MW01110379

ALSO BY CHRISTOPHER RAPPOLD

Be Your Personal Best: FOCUS

Be Your Personal Best: CONFIDENCE

How to Handle the Bully at School: A Parent's Guide

WARRIOR: A Tribute to Kevin Thompson, The Greatest Sport Martial Artist of All Time

Be Your Personal Best

FITNESS

CHRISTOPHER RAPPOLD

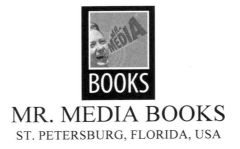

MR. MEDIA BOOKS
ST. PETERSBURG, FLORIDA, USA

ISBN-13: 978-1540747341

ISBN-10: 1540747344

Published by Mr. Media Books, St. Petersburg, Florida

For information, contact the author:
founder@personalbestkarate.com

To order additional print copies of
Be Your Personal Best: Fitness
Be Your Personal Best: Focus
Be Your Personal Best: Confidence
Please visit http://www.MrMediaBooks.com

Front and Back Cover Design by Lori Parsells
http://www.VibranceAndVision.com

To all the people who have taken the time to share their health and fitness wisdom with me, I offer this book as a way to pay it forward for the benefits I have received.

And for everyone who has ever felt confused, frustrated or dissatisfied with their level of health and fitness, this book is for you.

CONTENTS

"The investments we make in ourselves will always deliver the most profitable returns."
— *Sumner Davenport*

1. THE ULTIMATE LEVERAGE FOR LIFE: INVEST $4, GET BACK $96

How good does that sound to you? Do the math; it is a 24000% return!! Imagine going to Las Vegas with those odds in your favor. I don't think they would have the money left to build anymore big resorts. What about investing money in the stock market? You invest $4 and you get back $96, again a 24000% return! Won't be to long before you are purchasing a second home and an island to put it on. When we think in terms of examples like these, it is clear to see the power of the investment.

But when you talk about investing 4% of our day (1 hour) to give yourself the other 96% (23 hours) of being more productive, less stressed and able to enjoy a deeper more restful sleep, some will still turn away sighting everything from, "I don't have enough time" to "It's just not for me."

How can it be that on one hand someone understands the math but fails to make the connection? Well, I'm not sure I have the answer to that question but I do hope I see the shine of light bulb above your head because maybe for the first time you see how it can benefit you.

If Your "Why" Doesn't Make You Cry, It's *Not* Your "Why"!

2. WHY IS IT IMPORTANT TO YOU?

I am sure you have heard about the story of the grandmother lifting an end of a car up to free her trapped grandchild underneath it. How about the story of Marcus Luttrell, the Navy Seal who was shot several times, fell down a rocky cliff breaking his leg and his back, yet summoned the strength to crawl inch by inch seven miles to escape being captured? How is it that people are able to do these feats of what seems like impossibility?

I believe the reason is that their "why" is so strong that nothing will get in the way. For the grandmother, her "why" was the life of her grandchild and for Marcus Luttrell it was for his fellow Navy Seals and the love of his country. Though the examples are extreme, I think they both illustrate a point: when the "why" is strong enough, the excuses tend to fall aside.

So, let's bring it back to you. Living disease-free, being the best you that you can be, having more energy, being more productive and less stressed --are they enough motivation for you? For some, it is; for others, it still falls short.

I come from a belief that humans will always do more for others than they will for themselves. So if personal gain isn't enough, consider for a moment how you affect the people in your life that you love. Do you want to only be a fraction of what you could be as a wife or husband? How about as a parent: do you feel your children deserve the best parent they can possibly have or is a fraction of what you could be enough to give them? How about as a friend: is it important for you to have the energy and enthusiasm to be the very best friend you can be or, again, is good enough truly good enough? How about your career: is being a marginal version of yourself okay, knowing that you will ultimately be providing less for your family and that you will be competing against others who pride themselves in being the best they can be?

Self-investment is one of the single most impactful things you can possibly do for the people in your life. Think you are already doing a good enough job? Compared to what... the people around you? **Success is not measured by what you do compared to others; success is a personal measurement of how good you do, compared to how good you could have done maximizing all the abilities given to you.**

Perhaps the place to start first is with a list of the top 10 reasons taking better care of yourself physically, mentally emotionally and spiritually is important to you. With strong enough reasons for making the emotional commitment to a small investment of 4% you will have enjoy all the benefits of a 24000% return. Invest the time to put a list of the top ten most compelling reasons you will commit to it and keep this list in your office, in your car, on your desktop, on your phone - always in plain site as a way to keep you coming from a place of total commitment. A strong enough list of "whys" will always win over the tendency to not follow through.

"If you want to go fast, go alone. If you want to go far, go together."

— African Proverb

3. THE SINGLE MOST IMPORTANT DECISION FOR YOUR HEALTH AND FITNESS

There was a study done which focused on the most important factor in determining your health and fitness five years from today. Having a degree in Exercise Physiology, I wondered why they would research a question that had such a simple answer. Clearly the most important factor in determining health and fitness five years from today came down to your consistency to an exercise program. To my surprise… wrong! Well, clearly if it isn't exercise, then it must be the other major factor that people tend to stumble on, nutrition. Once again… wrong!

At this point I have to admit I was skeptical. Studying four years in college taught me that the combination of exercise and nutrition was the key to health and fitness. How could it be anything but your input – what you eat or output – your exercise program?

When I heard the answer I realized that what college did not teach me in its pursuit of a scientific answer, life outside of school had already taught me. The most important factor determining your health and fitness five years from today came down to the people in your immediate social circle.

I thought about it and just how important it was. When you hang out with friends who are always going out for pizza and beer where do you think you will be spending your time? When you hang out with friends who spend their nights on Facebook posting the best TV shows to watch, do you think you will be on a treadmill or on the couch? When you hang out with friends who live by the saying, "I'm here for a good time, not a long time" what do you think your habits will be?

Contrast that with a close peer group who is very conscious of making healthy food choices, prioritizing a regular exercise program that fits nicely into their daily routine and priding themselves on living a healthy disease free life.

Yes, it's true! As you start your journey, set yourself up for success by taking an open honest look at the people who surround you. Are their habits consistent with the personal goals you have for yourself? If not, beware! Maybe it's time to balance your time with some different people in your peer group so that you can enjoy the reminders and momentum from people who are on the same journey as you.

"You need to overcome the tug of people against you as you reach for higher goals."
— General George S. Patton

4. WHO IS AGAINST YOU?

No one is against you, right? Well, I think you will be surprised. Negative thinking? Not really. I just want you to be prepared for what at times may feel like a tidal wave of momentum testing your resolve.

Let's start with all the organizations whose best interest isn't in keeping you healthy. To get the impact of how many there are, take two days and keep track of all the commercials you see on TV. Ask yourself, "If I patronize their business, is it going to help me get healthy?" Next, while you are driving around start to do the same. Notice all the businesses that occupy the most heavily traffic areas. It's not your fault. You are barraged with continual advertisements that are designed to lure you in to patronize their establishments.

Want to take your family to a football, baseball, basketball game, who is present trying to steal your attention. What about taking your children to the movies or to the circus? What is right there waiting to tempt you? How about going into the grocery store, take a close look what is on both sides of you as you go to check out. Are you getting the idea? Temptation from huge corporations is all around. Know this, prepare for it and instead of giving into it take pride in being immune to it. Every time you pass on the temptation of giving those companies more money you are casting a vote for yourself.

What about your family and friends? Do they love you...absolutely!

Will they be happy and supportive of the changes you make? It depends on whether they share a healthy consistent lifestyle that you are going for. If they are not, know that resistance may come in the form of lots of unintentional comments made for your new nutritional choices and how you are spending your time. It is not done with mean intentions, but the human side of it is when family and friends feel you changing your habits that are the entwined sources that bond you together, understandably they may try to poke holes in your efforts.

Prepare for this and at the start, ask them for their support and why it is important for you to make the changes. Be prepared to continue to remind them as well. In most cases, if you approach it correctly, you will find they will share your enthusiasm. Who knows, maybe you can bring some along with them on your journey for a healthy energetic lifestyle.

It takes 4 weeks for you to see your body changing.

It takes 8 weeks for your family and friends to notice.

It takes 12 weeks for the world to see the change in you.

KEEP GOING!

5. WHAT IS YOUR STARTING POINT?

When you begin an exercise and nutrition program much of your motivation to continue and all of your adjustments will come from the accurate feedback you receive. That being said, knowing exactly where you are starting from becomes a critical component to your long-term success.

Most people begin a program and take the approach of jumping on a scale to see how much they weigh. Makes sense, right? Well, I can tell you the scale can be your greatest source of discouragement. Let me tell you why.

Whatever your weight, the number only represents the total amount of pounds. While this number is accurate, it only tells a portion of the story. Imagine for a moment two different people each weigh themselves and they both tip the scales at 200 pounds. One of these people was a male body builder and the other a sedentary couch potato. How could it be the scale said the same thing? Because the scale accurately measures only one thing: weight. It gives no indication of whether it is measuring 200 pounds of rocks or 200 pounds of chocolate.

We have had many a student at Personal Best Karate get on a scale and feel discouraged because their weight wasn't moving, even though they could tell their clothes were fitting differently. Immediately they assumed they were failing, until we revealed to them what was being measured. Think for a moment the shift in motivation when a female student whose weight hadn't changed but then learns she lost 3% of her body fat and gained 1% in muscle... What a difference in motivation! She goes from a feeling of, "No matter what I try, it doesn't work" to "Hey, I can do this!" Though she was winning, if she only looked at the weight she may get discouraged and quit, never knowing the improvements that were being made.

One of the best things you can do for yourself is get a body composition test done at the start of your training. No matter what the score, the only thing you are concerned with is that in two weeks when you have it done again, your fat percentage is decreasing and muscle percentage in increasing... success at last!

Yesterday, you said, "Tomorrow."

START NOW!

6. WHEN DO YOU START?

I think I am going to start right in the New Year.

I am going to start once the kids are back in school.

I'm going to start as soon as the kids get out of school.

I'm going to start once the project at work is done.

I'm going to start as soon as my knee feels better.

I'm going to start as soon as I can get my friend to go to the gym with me.

Do any of these phrases sound familiar? Have your ever heard someone else say one of these or have you ever had one of these thoughts in your head? Recognize them for what they are… procrastination disguised in social acceptable excuses.

The fact is, life happens to us all. Urgency in health and fitness only happens when you get the disease, have the heart attack or develop Type 2 diabetes. Other than that, the decision will never be urgent but it is always extremely important. So when should you start? You should start today! No matter what!

Nutritional food choices can happen with your next meal. Exercise can happen within your next five minutes of free time. How long does it take you to run in place for 30 seconds, do 10 squats, 10 push ups, 10 sit ups and a sit and reach stretch? Time needn't be a limiting factor in delaying you taking a step towards a better healthier and fit you. Remind yourself, whenever you are tempted to fall into the trap of reasoning why you can't all you are doing is making an excuse that with a little thought you would be able to easily leap frog over.

Progress?

You might not be where you want to be, but you aren't where you used to be.

7. HOW DO YOU MEASURE PROGRESS?

How you measure your progress will make a big difference in your ability to create momentum and create the understanding you need so that you are in control of your body. They saying, "What gets measured can be managed" is truer that perhaps you even realize when it comes to fitness.

Without clear guideline measurements, you will understandably fall in the trap of comparing your progress to the people around you. Most of the time this will not be motivating due to many people's self critical nature. Sometimes people will compare themselves to the people they see on television or in magazines, not realizing that many of the photos have been enhanced to provide an almost unattainable physique. Feeling like you can never hit the goal, eventually you simply decide to give in and quit.

As a defense to the above temptations, let's set you up by success by giving you some tangible measurements that are meaningful. To do this, start with the pledge that you will only compare yourself to your previous results. For example, if you choose to check in each month and measure your blood pressure, you only compare it to your previous score, not your friend's blood pressure. If you are measuring your waist, it is only compared to your previous score.

Some reasonable suggestions of things that would be good to

measure:

• Blood Pressure: particularly recommended if your doctor sites this as a concern for you.

• Cholesterol: recommended if your doctor sites this as a concern for you.

• Body Composition (lean muscle compared to fat)

• Body measurements including circumferences of stomach, waist, hips, thighs, calves chest, arms. Measuring each site will give you an indication if the desired outcome is being met. Sometimes someone who only measures one site such as waist will become discouraged never realizing the difference in their arm measurement. Everyone's body is different. Some will lose it in different places first which is why multiple sites are recommended.

• Daily perceive energy: this can be self-estimated on a scale of 1 -10 each day. You want to see the numbers over time become consistently higher. This gives you an indication that your exercise and nutritional program is working to enhance your daily life.

While there is no concrete rule as to how often you should measure, I think in the beginning once every two weeks is long enough to show progress yet short enough to keep you motivated and in tune with your fitness and nutrition program.

"Simplicity: Identify the essential. Eliminate the rest."
— Leo Babauta

8. SIMPLY THEN PROCESS: DESIGN AN AUTOMATED PLAN

It is much better to start on the shoulders of people who are experts in fitness and nutrition especially in the beginning of your fitness journey. So many times a person is filled with the motivation to finally, at long last, get in shape only to be discouraged and frustrated by a lack of progress. Think about it: would you ever decide to start investing money into the stock market without knowing how? Of course not! But every day, well-intentioned people make the mistake of getting started without the know how of how to proceed.

Instead of going at it alone decide to give yourself the advantage of automating the what and when: what exercises should you be doing and for how long, and when will this routine happen in your week. This will help you in not being weighed down by a ton of decisions that you don't have the answers to; rather, all you have to do is show up to the program the number of days selected and simply follow the plan.

Many times I hear people say, "If I just knew what to do, I would do it." By choosing this approach you have peace of mind to know that the protocol laid before you has been designed and proven to produce your desired outcome. A word of caution: make sure the facility you place your trust in is clean, well-maintained, has a culture that supports your goals and has a track record of producing results.

"Our food should be our medicine and our medicine should be our food."

— Hippocrates

9. CHANGE NUTRITION HABITS ONE DAY AT A TIME

Correct nutrition is one of those things that have a major effect on virtually every area of your life. Wherever you go, whomever you are with, and whatever you are doing throughout the course of a day, what you are eating follows you. Whether at a wedding or working out in the yard, in traffic or on a tropical island, nutrition is interwoven into your day. It stands to reason that what you are putting into your body will have a major impact on your energy.

Dr. Mark Mincolla, a brilliant holistic doctor (MarkMincolla.com) teaches the concept of the food we eat as natural medicine. There are foods that heal and there are foods that cause inflammation in our bodies. There are foods that provide vital nutrients and foods that leach nutrients from our body. There are foods that build and there are foods that destroy. Taking the time to analyze the impact of what you are putting into your body is a worthy study that will quite literally add years of good health to your life. As you delve into the topic you will learn that every body has a different chemistry and what is good for one person may not be good for another. Like a fingerprint, each person is unique and different and needs to be respected as such. Learning it yourself or finding an expert like Dr. Mincolla is certainly a shortcut to making this happen for you.

Here are habits in install and maintain to provide better nutritional choices. They are simple to understand and will aid in helping you be a better you. Don't try to change them all at once; changing them one day at a time will ensure they stick.

Here are the Best Habits to Establish and Maintain

Water: So many people unknowingly walk around at a significant disadvantage of being continually dehydrated. As a general rule, aim to drink half your body weight in ounces of water each day. This will provide you with the necessary fluids to think more clearly, and allow your body to function optimally. As you create this habit, be sure that water is in its purest form, you cannot count consumption of coffee, tea, soda or alcoholic beverages.

Water Rich Foods: What percentage of each meal is made up of vegetables? Most would agree that 50 – 75% of every meal you consume should consist of vegetables or legumes. If you look at the average American diet it is completely reversed. 25% is green and 75% is non-water rich like chicken or steak.

Eat smaller portions: Think about how you feel at the end of your Thanksgiving meal. Bloated, sluggish and generally craving a nap. Digestion is the largest energy drain placed on our body. Instead of eating three large meals per day, which will contribute to you feeling fatigued, think about eating six smaller meals per day; grazing instead of gorging. An indicator if you are eating correctly is how you feel immediately after you eat. If you are feeling tired perhaps you are putting too much demand on your body all at once.

Honor the Three Hour Rule: As mentioned previously, digestion is the biggest drain on your physical body. It stands to reason, that when you eat prior to going to bed, your physical body will be up working hard to digest what was consumed instead of enjoying a vital recharge. If you are going to bed each evening at 10 p.m., then plan your last meal to be no later than 7 p.m. By creating this you allow digestion to occur during waking hours instead of sleeping hours.

Read the labels: You don't have to be an expert. A simple rule of thumb is if you don't recognize the word, can't pronounce it or have no idea what it is, then don't eat the food. This will significantly alter what you are putting into your body by keeping you eating only foods that can feed your body with the right kind of nutrients.

Here are a couple quick ways to weed out other foods that you should eliminate as a regular part of your nutritional plan. If a food has 15 grams of sugar or less, 200mg of salt or less and 25% of calories or less from fat then it is a go. If it breaks any of the above three rules then you eliminate it as a part of your regular daily plan.

Personal Best Guide to Eating Healthy

Personal Planning is key to ensuring your newly acquired knowledge is applied. To help with this take the time to fill out a few different versions of a daily nutritional plan that allows you to follow the advice given. By taking the time to write it down, you are ensuring your shopping will support your goals and that you can now set your eating habits on automatic pilot.

Breakfast

Mid morning snack

Lunch

Mid afternoon snack

Dinner

Early evening snack

<u>Flawsome</u> *(adj.)*: **An individual who embraces his flaws and knows he is awesome, regardless.**

10. HOPE FOR THE BEST BUT PREPARE FOR IMPERFECTION

Imagine you just finished reading this book. For the fist time, you feel a sense of clarity about what you need to do to give yourself the body and the energy you deserve. The next day you are invited to a family member's birthday party and you indulge in a piece of birthday cake. Immediately you feel the guilt of not sticking with your plan. As you embark on this plan, know in advance that to achieve your goal you do not have to be perfect, just very consistent. There will be times through no fault of your own you will have to be less than perfect. Imagine you are invited over a friend's house and they have spent all day preparing a meal, but the meal is filled with high fat content foods. You don't want to offend your friend so you enjoy the meal along with them. Imagine you are traveling and the airport you land after a six-hour flight only has fast food, you do your best but know that it wasn't perfect.

While some of these situations may be prevented with some advanced planning, let me assure you not all can be nor should all be avoided. After all what kind of life do you have when your nutrition is so restrictive that you can't enjoy a piece of cake birthday celebration?

The most important decision that needs to be made is that if there is a cheat meal or a cheat day, that you are right back on the plan the next day. Avoid letting a cheat turn into a gateway of unrestricted eating.

So what are some ways you can prevent your nutrition from getting away from you.

If you going out to eat, decide in advance that you are going to be eating a big salad and asking for a double vegetable. This will assure you maintain the 50 -75% rule of water rich foods.

If you have a day that you will be traveling, instead of being at the mercy of what is around you, plan on bringing healthy snacks, like fruit and cut up vegetables with you. Also plan on bringing enough water to keep you adequately hydrated.

If you are going to be dining at someone else's home enjoy whatever they have made but bias the portion of what you are eating and do your best to fill your plate with the best food choices available.

If you are going to a holiday party or a place that you know will have a lot of dessert options, decide in advance the quantity you will have. If you want to sample a few different desserts then think about taking small portions so that you can enjoy without feeling like you cheated your cheat meal.

These are a few strategies that have worked to allow you to keep on track despite the nutritional distractions that will naturally occur. The idea is, with a little planning you can have your cake and eat it too.

Bonus: A Sweet, Healthy Treat!

Take 1 cup of cooked fruit after dinner each night! Fill a Pyrex container with frozen berries, unsweetened canned peaches and pears. Add cinnamon, and oatmeal flakes. Bake at 350 degrees for 50 minutes. Over the past 25 years my patients have reported that this pie filling like dessert satisfies their sweet tooth in a most healthy way! — *Dr. Mark Mincolla*

Push harder than yesterday if you want a different tomorrow.

11. FITNESS MADE SIMPLE

Like all things, you can make it as complicated or simple to follow as possible. You don't need a huge amount of time, expensive equipment or a PhD in Exercise Physiology to enjoy a healthy active lifestyle. When you reduce fitness down to its major elements you will find it includes strength, endurance and flexibility. Now there are thousands of different ways to improve each of the three based on an individual's access to knowledge and exercise preferences, but all roads applied consistently will lead to an improved result.

Strength: To simplify strength, we can look at lower body, middle body also referred to as "core" and upper body. To add strength to each part you want to start with four core exercises. For upper body: pull-ups and push-ups. For Core: sit-ups and back extensions. For lower: body squats and lunges. For each of these exercises you can conveniently find how to correctly perform each via a YouTube video.

To start your exercise program simply get a baseline measurement of what you can do and plan to increase your activity by concentrating on these six exercises two– three times per week. Keep track of your progress by counting the number of repetitions you are able to do. Once you are able to complete ten with great form then increase to a second set of each exercise.

Endurance: For endurance, the easiest way to start to increase your endurance is to start with walking. Plan on investing ten minute per day. Once your able to satisfy this minimum starting point then you follow suit by increasing either the pace: turning your walk into a jog, time: 10 minutes to 20 minutes or distance one mile to two miles. In whichever measurement feels right to your body, the most important consideration is consistency. Keeping a daily routine of endurance, which exercises your heart will start to slowly but surely give you more energy.

Flexibility: The final consideration to a well-rounded exercise program is flexibility. Keeping your muscles flexibility improves your performance and decreases your risk of injuries by helping your joints move through their full range of motion. This in turn enables your muscles to work most effectively. Like with strength, you want to ensure upper, core and lower body flexibility. To gain the most effective benefit it is widely accepted to stretch after your body temperature is heated by a warm up or by a complete exercise session. Saving flexibility improvement for the end of your workout period and holding each stretch statically for a minimum of 30 seconds seems to give the best result.

For the legs, picking and stretching for your quads, hamstrings, abductors and adductors and calves should give you a good start.

For the core of your body you want to pick a stretch that stretches your lower back stomach and oblique muscles.

For your upper body, simple stretches that address upper back flexibility, shoulders and chest and neck is a great place to start.

As with strength exercises, if you enter stretches for and you add a body part you will be treated to many YouTube videos that show exactly the movements you need to start enjoying the benefits of greater flexibility. When you find the exercises be sure to write them down and follow the correct form of each.

The above exercise recommendation takes the approach of creating a way for you to start a self-paced program that will benefit you if you are planning to workout on your own. If you would rather join a program and follow the close advice and council of experts in health and fitness you can very easily attend your class two to four times per week and get all the benefits without having to construct a program from start to finish. In either case, consistency over time wins the day.

Surround yourself with those who *challenge* you, *push* you, *know* you, and *motivate* you to be your personal best!

12. CHOOSE A FITNESS PROGRAM THAT IS RIGHT FOR YOU!

If you are looking for a program to invest your time and energy into you want to be sure that you meet and exceed your expectations. Let's face it, if you pay $50 on a program and it doesn't give the result you want most would say you wasted your money. However, if you spent $300 on a program that helped guide you to find the strength and endurance and flexibility that you always wanted most would say that was well worth it.

As person who has trained alongside hundreds of martial artists and fitness enthusiasts over my adult life, I have had the chance to see first hand both successful and unsuccessful programs. The following is a list of criteria I would suggest you use as you evaluate and find a program that meets your needs and can deliver on your hopes and dreams.

Enthusiasm of the teachers: Many fitness enthusiasts are self-focused. A criterion they use to enroll you in their program is to talk about themselves. Not that they are bad people but their tendency is to serve their ego rather than serve their students. I love to see a teacher who gets excited about the progress of their students because she knows the importance of what it means to them. When you are trained by a person or a team that enthusiastically cheers you on and transfers that joy to you each and every time, it ensures that you stay inspired to continue to make progress.

Program Longevity and Results Produced: The quality of a program's success should rest on the results the students have attained. Are the people in the program getting the results and has the teaching team been doing it long enough that they have the depth of experience to know how to work with all different populations? I have seen a lot of programs come and go like the changing of the tides. What is hot today is gone tomorrow. If you are in this for the lifestyle take careful consideration in choosing the program that is right for you.

Facility cleanliness: I believe this is very important in a student's overall success. Air quality, cleanliness of the equipment being used and continued maintenance shows that the teacher and team are attentive to details and values the students or clients at a high level. When you are sweating and working hard you don't want the distractions of sweat stains, offensive odor or unsafe equipment being used. Facilities should be cleaned regularly to ensure the highest experience.

Training Routine and Curriculum: The curriculum should be easy to follow, safe for the participants and allow for accountability of progress. You are enrolling for a reason, while there are no guarantees in life; you want to stack the deck in your favor. If the curriculum is easy to follow that translates to certainty and predictability. The last thing you want to have happen while you are making efforts to enhance your life is a needless injury that sidelines you. A program that was thoughtfully assembled with students like you in mind can make all the difference in the world. If you are a forty five year old women and the class curriculum gears itself to 22-year-old male athletes approach, as competent as the instructors may be it will be a mismatch. An easy way to assess this is to view a class. See if with reasonable effort you could acclimate yourself into the training.

Your Training Partners: The people involved with the training create the culture. Are you looking for a militant fear based training program where the competitive nature of the training involved creates progress or do you prefer a welcoming environment where everyone encourages each other and realizes they are all part of the same team? Nothing is right or wrong it is just what do you prefer. Again you will get a sense of this by watching or participating in a class.

13. FINAL THOUGHTS

Everyone deserves to experience the feeling of being at his or her best. A big part of that comes from what we eat, how we take care of our bodies and most importantly who we spend most of our time with. Having energy makes life so much easier and now I hope you understand how to crack the code of your own fitness lifestyle. When you install healthy routines and habits you set yourself up for a great day and an even better long- term healthy life. It is well within all of our control.

If you read this book to start on the journey of an improved fitness lifestyle, I hope you got some great gems that you can put to use immediately. If you were reading this so you can share improve the health and fitness of your family I commend you on your commitment to invest the time to learn implement and share the lifelong value gained from a healthy lifestyle. I hope you are able to take and use this book to start the journey of being a more healthy you.

KEEP THE MOMENTUM FROM THIS BOOK GOING STRONG!

ABOUT THE AUTHOR
CHRISTOPHER M. RAPPOLD

Christopher Rappold is a master teacher, trainer and blogger who has been working with children and families for more than 25 years. He has presented bullying programs to more than 30 school districts and is a widely recognized expert at presenting safety strategies and bullying prevention in layman's terms while also filling gaps left by educating and involving teachers, parents and school administrators.

Rappold is the founder of Personal Best Karate, martial arts schools presently located in New England, and serves as both an owner and president of the franchise. His form of teaching honors the potential of each student's individual capabilities and works to ensure just the right level of challenge is presented so that the student can maintain sustained and lasting growth and improvement.

Rappold has been a member of Team Paul Mitchell (the top-rated sport karate team in the world) dating back to 1988 and currently serves as the team's Executive Director. Rappold has also won the W.A.K.O. World Championship in three different weight divisions.

Training at Personal Best Karate is a great way to bring a steady practice of fitness into your family's life. Please consider accepting the gift of a FREE trial in our award-winning character-based martial arts or kickboxing program. We pride ourselves in being experts in developing mental and physical skills to help our students realize their fullest potential.

Please go to www.PersonalBestKarate.com.

We promise that our team of highly skilled martial arts teachers and mentors will help you and your family feel right at home.

For more information on Personal Best Karate programs, or to gift yourself or someone you know with a free trial, please call (508) 285-5425 or email info@personalbestkarate.com.